The WEB SPINNERS

Editor in Chief
Dr. Farokh J. Master

Asst. Editors
Dr. Renuka D. Punjabi
Dr. Pranesh R. Shroff
Dr. Ronak J. Shah
Dr. Sanjay Shah
Dr. Piroja M. Bharucha

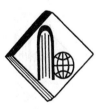

B. JAIN PUBLISHERS (P) Ltd.

First Edition 1995
Reprint Edition : 1997, 2002, 2004

Price : Rs. 29.00

© Copyright with Publishers

Published by:
B. Jain Publishers (P) Ltd.
1921, Street No. 10th Chuna Mandi,
Paharganj, New Delhi-110055 (INDIA)

Phones: 2358 0800, 2358 1100, 2358 1300, 2358 3100
Fax: 011-2358 0471   *Email:* bjain@vsnl.com
Website: **www.bjainbooks.com**

Printed in India by :
J.J. Offset Printers

Cover page Designed by :
        Mr. Dara Ichhaporia,
        M/s Dara Designing Concepts,
        Colsawala Building, Cowasji Patel Street,
        Fort, Bombay-400001

ISBN-81-7021-578-1

Book Code BM-5126

INDEX

FOREWORD

In this compilation "Spiders" are presented in the form of a small animated picture.

In addition to the individual characteristics, I have discovered the properties of various spider poisons which I have used to bring about some wonderful recoveries.

May this compilation lead to ever greater enthusiasm on the part of the doctor of homoeopathy everywhere as they strive to increase their knowlege.

I would consider my labour amply rewarded if this compilation succeeds in maintaining its tradition and reputation of being styled as a pocket compilation of individual Materia Medica in the truest sense of the term.

I would fail to perform my duty if I do not mention the name of Mr. Kuldeep Jain who has always encouraged my endeavours. I would also like to metion my friend, Mr. Dara Ichhaporia who so artistically designs the cover page of my various publication. Last but not the least, my sincere thanks to Miss Roda Bandrawala, Mrs. Aloo Irani for typing the manuscripts.

Dr. Farokh J. Master

19th Nov. 1994.

DEDICATION

This book is dedicated to
Dr. Premnath Jain
Mr. Kuldeep Jain
Mr. Ashok Jain

The three pillars of M/s. B. Jain Homoeopathic
Publication who have put India in the
map of the World as the largest
publication company in
homoeopathic
field.

SALUTATIONS

My assistants as usual have laboured to find reference works as well as bear my moods during the preparation of my compilation.

My sincere thanks to :

Dr. Kamal Kodia

Dr. Kamal Rustomjee

Dr. Benaz Marolia

Dr. Niloufer N. Bamji

Dr. Diana Minbattiwala

Dr. Kehkashan Deshmukh

Dr. Afshan Deshmukh

Dr. Zenobia Colabawalla

Dr. Binal Shah

Dr. Amisha Bangdiwala

Dr. Sangeeta Pooran

Dr. Shailen Petigara

Dr. Shahrukh K.R. Pavri

Dr. Zubin Marolia

Dr. Paresh Thakkar

Dr. Rohit Sharma

Dr. Pratik Maniar

Dr. R.S. Yadav

Dr. Meena Goshar

Dr. Priya Panchal

Dr. Uma Chaudhry

Dr. Chetna Thakkar

SPIDERS

Spiders from the largest and most widely distributed order of class of animals called ARACHNIDA, which also includes the scorpions, hervestmen, false scorpions, mites and ticks.

There are about 22,000 different species of spiders of which about 500 are British. The largest are found in Central America and have a body length of about 3.5 inches, the smallest species are less than a 25th of an inch long.

SPIDERS - ARANEIDA

There are two types of spiders :

1. ARANOMORPHAE or DIPNEUMONES, with one pair of lungs.

2. MYGALOMORPHAE or TETRAPNEUMONES, with two pairs of lungs.

ARANOMORPHAE

1. They spin cobwebs in the air.

MYGALOMORPHAE

1. Always live in funnels and tubular holes in the ground. Some close this beutifully lined holes with a lid like a hinge door.

2. The poison glands and ducts are elongated and the claws move horizontally like pin	2. They have short glands and ducts and their fangs move vertically.
3. Tarentula Hispanica	3. Tarentula Cubensis Mygale Cubensis

More species belong to the Aranomorphae and they are called the true spiders or tarentulas (in the new nomenclature tarantula).

Bodies of animals belonging to class Arachnida - consist of 2 parts :

(a) The front - head and chest closely joined forming cephalothorax;

(b) The behind - the abdomen.

Greek Mythology

In ancient Greece there lived a woman called Arachne who was famous for her skill in weaving. Her skill at her art made her very conceited, thinking that there was none better than her. In her conceit she challenged the Goddess Athene to a weaving contest. Arachne's effort was very beautiful and it aroused jealousy in Athene was felt threatened by Arachne. Athene was the goddess of all weaving. In her fit of rage she tore Arachne's wearing to pieces. Arachne was very upset and she hung herself, where upon Athene changed her into a spider and condemned her to go on weaving forever. Hence, the name Arachnida which really means "Children of Arachne".

The have a pair of jaws, a pair of pincer claws and

4 pairs of legs, all attached to the cephalothorax.

Above features and lack of antennae distinguish the arachnida from insects.

As exclusive predators, the spiders have invented a number of cunning stratagies for catching their food. Many, like the wolf spiders are active hunters. They are swift runners and have large eyes - so they can seek out and run down their prey. Spiders secrete silk through six tubular spinnerets, placed at the tip of the abdomen. The silk is then used to spin the web.

Spiders have an extremely delicate sence of touch whcih enables them to detct their prey by the vibrations of the threads of their silk webs. When spiders bite, they paralyse their victims with poison secreted from glands in their jaws.

Poison is injected by means of a pair of hollow fangs, so that the spider can be said to stab rather than sting or bite. Its mouthparts are designed for sucking up the juices of its prey, it cannot chew solid food and the victim is eventually discarded as a dry husk.

The spider's fangs are like the teeth of a lion or the fangs of a snake. If the predator itself is in danger, it can turn its weapons on its attacker.

The venom has an effect on such small animals as mice, moles and sparrows - but only a few spiders are dangerous to man.

Some large species have fangs - long and strong enough to penetrate the human skin. One such is the baboon spider of Africa.

The symptoms of spider bite are unpleasant. The venom is a neurotoxin which causes paralysis, muscular cramp and severe pain. Breathing becomes difficult and the victim runs a high fever.

Reaction to venom varies from individual to individual. Some people are extremely sensitive and can suffer severely or even die from a single sting.

Spiders share a common habit of trailing behind them a dragline of silk, fastened at intervals. If the spider misses its footing, the drag-line, like a mountaineer's rope, saves it from falling to the ground.

Their habits vary in the peculiar methods of courtship in different families. When a male spider visits a female spider, to mate with her, he plucks the mating, the male spider usually escapes at his best speed. The belief that female spiders always eat their mates - is an exaggeration - exception being towards the end of autumn when females are likely to be hungry and the males less active.

All spiders start life as eggs, usually laid in masses in a silk cocoon. Generally, the female pays little attention to her cocoon after it is completed. Spiders do not go through a larval stage - but resemble their parents when they hatch. They grow by periodic castings of their skin. The sex of the spider is usually impossible to tell until it is mature.

'Gossamer' is produced by young spiders of many species and by adults of a few, in their peculiar method of migration. When the weather is suitable, they climb up fences and railings, turn their heads towards the wind, raise their abdomens and exude silk. The drop of silk is drawn out by the breeze into a long thread and when sufficient buoyancy is attained, the spider lets go and drifts away.

· The strangest trick af all is used by certain spiders which have no web but spin a single thread with a stickly blob at the end. This is whirled, until it `hooks' an insect.

Crab spiders walk sideways in the same way as crabs. They can change colour to match their hiding places, and they lie in ambush for small insects inside flowers or among leaves. Their popular name is descriptive, for they are flattened in from with crab-like legs and a habit of darting sideways.

The small brown spiders of woods and greenlands called **wolf spiders** - run fast enough to pursue their quary and overtake it. The wolf spider waves his decorated forelegs in front of the female during the mating - as a habit peculiar to the Wolf spiders. They fasten their cocoons onto themselves and carry them about till the hatch. Then for a time, the baby spiders ride on their mother's back.

The black & white **jumping spiders** have better eyesight than other spiders. They stalk insects, creeping along tree trunks and old walls; towards their prey, as a cat stalks a mouse, and then leaping on it. Before jumping, they spin out a lifeline of silk, fastening one end of it to the bark or the wall, so that if they miss a fall, they can climb back to safety. The male jumping spider performs a kind of dance in front of the watching female.

The perfection of web-spinning is found in the cartwheel or orb-web spun by the Garden Spider and other members of its family. Argyopidae. To make a web, the

Garden Spider, first fastens four threads of silk among leaves or on brickwork to form a square, across which it stretches other threads to meet in the middle, like the spokes of a wheel. Next, it lays down a thread of silk in a spiral, which it fastens to the spokes, wherever they cross. This is a temporary web, which gives the spider something to walk on while spinning the real one. The spider now spins a very sticky kind of silk, with which it builds the real web. As it lays down each piece of this from the outside to the centre, it cuts away a piece of the temporary web and swallows it.

The **net casting** spider uses a stranger stratagem to trap its prey. The web is stretched between the spider's legs and is used to sweep up passing insects.

The **purse** spiders spin a tube that lies on the ground and connects with a tunnel. When an insect walks over the tube, the spider seizes it with its fangs, cuts a slit in the silk and hauls the victim in.

The giant **Bird-eating spider,** an inhabitant of the Amazon jungle, which can consume small humming birds, is a rather inoffensive animal. The hazard from handling it is irritation from the hairs, and it may threaten its foes by raising its forelegs (like the baboon spider). By day, it hides in rock crevices, under loose bark or in a hollow tree where it rests on a pad of silk. It spins no web but runs down its prey in a silent pounce. As soon as such a prey is seized, it is stabbed by the fangs and injected with a lethal dose of venom.

The **baboon spider,** lives in burrows. Its bite, although painful, has an effect less than that of a wasp sting. This spider plays a beneficial role of eating army worms - the destructive moth caterpillars which devour grass, as locusts devour leaves.

The **Brazilian huntsman spider,** is another large species capable of delivering a venomous bite. It captures its prey by running it down. Eyesight is more important to this agile creature than to the web spinners.

The **thorn spider** is a South American species, but similar spiny bodied spiders are found through out the tropics. They are usually small, but conspicuous because of their bright, warning colors, usually black with red and yellow. They are not known to be poisonous to man.

The large **Trap-door** Spiders of the tropics, live in a silk-lined tunnel in the soil which is closed by a tightly-fitting - camouflaged lid, which serves as a trap door, and it is covered with earth. Silk trip wires radiate from the tube so that the spider knows the instant that some small animal wanders into the range. They raise the trap door to rush out at their victims, then retire into their burrow, closing the trap door behind them and devour their catch. They include the largest species known and sometimes misnamed tarentulas.

Perhaps, the most dangerous of all spiders is the Black Widow. It is found in many of the warmer parts of N. America. It appears innocuous - only half inch long with a shiny black body and no hairs. On the underside, there is a red mark in the perfect shape of an hourglass, which has earned the species the alternative names of hourglass spider and red mark. Though the Black Widow is a shy and retiring animal, it should be treated with caution as its venom is said to be 15 times more powerful than that of a rattlesnake. Its danger arises from the fact that it rushes out to investigate anything that vibrates its web and attacks everything - from a fly to the human finger. The web is built across a gap, where insects are likely to fly.

It is unfortunate that spiders should have such a poor reputation, because they do no harm and as insect eaters, they play an important part in wild life economy. Their habits also make them one of the most interesting groups of animals to study.

ARANEA DIADEMA

Source : The cross spider - this spider is not poisonous to human beings, but it is supposed to have a poison which kills birds - they die from cramps.

Proving : The first proving was done in 1832 by Grauvogl.

Symptomatology General : Neuralgic pains < menses > hard pressure. Haemorrhages from all organs. Feeling as if parts were enlarged or heavier. All symptoms are characterised by periodicty & coldness. Sensation of swelling of hands and forearms on waking.

Constitution : Constitutions favourable to malarial poisoning. Hydrogenoid constitution patient has abnormal sensitiveness to damp and cold. Cannot live near fresh water, lakes, rivers or in damp and chilly places.

Mind : Despondent; longs for death.

Head : Headache with burning of forehead and face, preceded by vertigo and flickering before eyes, cannot sit up - has to lie down.

Headache > smoking tobacco.
> open air.

Teeth : Pain in teeth < night, on lying down, cold feeling in teeth, which comes on peroidcally.

Mouth : Tongue - bitter taste with coated tongue > smoking, pain at root of tongue and in lower jaw. Tongue - alomost paralysed, utterance thick and heavy.

Stomach : Eating causes headache and spasms. Vomiting with fever. Epigastrium painful to pressure.

Abdomen : Enlarged spleen with chilliness. Fullness and heaviness in abodmen as if from a stone. Colic with shuddering towards evening. Diarhoea - watery with rumbling, with sensation as if arms and legs were asleep.

Female : Menses too early, profuse, long lasting. Metrorrhagia, bright red blood, Viscous leucorrhoea. Neuralgic pains (right sided) < during menses > hard pressure.

Respiratory Orgnas : Haemoptysis in anaemic and debilitated subjects.

Extremeties : Bone pains. Pain in Os Calcis - sensation of swelling and of parts going to sleep. Numbness of parts supplied by ulnar nerve.

Sleep : Restless with frequent waking; On waking some parts of the body feel swollen. Pain in teeth on lying down at night.

Fever : Before chill - cramps in abdomen, vomiting, backache; Chilly as if bones made of ice < rain. Chill with clock like periodicity. Chill everyday at the same hour. During chill - pains in head, stomach, knees. During heat - headache with drowsiness. After heat - vomiting prostration, lies as if dead. Sweat with or without thirst.

Modalities - < damp weather
              < at midnight,

< late in afternoon,
> smoking tobacco.

Clinical - Affections of bones. Haemorrhages. Chills, Dysmenorrhoea, Headache. Malaria, Neuralgia. Punctured wounds. Scorbutic affection. Scurvy. Rickets. Spleen. Affection. Toothache.

Relationship - Compare : Mygale, Theridion, Tarent., Ipec., Nux-v., Ars (intermittents and bone affections). Cedron (Intermittent of hot climates; Aranae - of cold climates).

Antidoted by smoking tobacco.

ARANEA DIADEMA

In my early practice, I used this remedy for Calcaneal spur based on the rubric given in the Kent's Repertory.

* Extremities - Pain, foot, heel.
* Extremities - Pain, joints.
* Extremities - Pain, boring heel.
* Extremities - Pain, boring os calcis, continued motion, amel.

I had once an occasion to observe late Dr. J. N. Kanjilal of Calcutta use this remedy for malarial fevers. During my residential A.M.O. post in the Homoeopathic hospital in the O.P.D., we saw a young Maharashtrian boy who had chronic Migraine which was better in open air. A characteristic symptom was, that the headache was better by smoking and worse on eating. On examination, there was an enlarged spleen. Few doses of Aranea in the 1M potency gradually helped to decrease his migraine which was of many years duration.

ARANEA SCINENCIA

Source : The source of this remedy is a grey spider found in Kentucky. This spider does not spin a web and is found on old walls.

Proving : Aranea Scinencia has been proved in 1st and 2nd dilutions. A very important symptom in the proving was constant twitching under eyelids.

Symptomatology :

Head : Dull, stupid headache especially in postero-superior part of head. Unable to rest. Feeling as if he was drunk.

Eyes : Inflammed, weak, watery, lids swollen, constant twitching under eyelids.

Mouth : Profuse flow of saliva. Sweet taste in the mouth.

Sleep : Sleepy feeling.

All symptoms are < in warm room.

Clinical : Debility

Eye affections.

Headache.

ARANEA TELA

Source : Cobweb of black spider found in barns, cellars and dark places.

This remedy has been used from ancient times.

Proving : During proving it was observed that this drug lowers the frequency of the pulse rate in healthy human beings. In some provers it produced a calm state of feeling, followed by a disposition to sleep.

Symptomatology :

Symptoms come on suddenly with cool, clammy skin.
Numbness of hands and legs when at rest.
Continued chilliness.
Masked periodical diseases, broken down patients.
Cardia sleeplessness, increased muscular energy.
Dry asthma, harassing cough.
Periodic headaches with extreme nervous erethism.
Obstinate intermittents.

Tela aranea was successfully used in a case of a middle aged woman who was diagnosed as a case of Supra Ventricular Tachycardia. Her constitutional remedy was selected as Calcarea ars. During the acute phase Digitalis, Gelsemium failed. Later Tela aranea was given on the following indications and she improved considerably :

* Rapid pulse rate.
* Weakness, want of energy.

It also calmed the patient with a feeling of tranquility.

LATRODECTUS MACTANS

Introduction :

Much has been written about Latrodecus Mactans consequences of its bite. This spider is found in South America and also inthe Southern States of North America.

Species :

Other species of Latrodectus are :

* Latrodectus tridecimguttatus - the Malmignatte of Southern Europe.
* Latrodectus lugubris - The Karakurt of Russia.
* Latrodectus hasselti - the Katipo of New Zealand.

Source/Pharmacognosy :

It is prepared from a small female spider of the Araneida family, which is rather obese and black all over except for a red or orange marking in the shape of an hour glass on the ventral aspect of the belly. The body of this full-grown female measures about half an inch in length and has eight one-inch long sprangling legs.

After mating, the femal eats the male, which is much smaller in size compared to the femal. Hence it is known as the "Black Widow Spider."

It fetters its prey which may be many times its own size and weight in a very strong mantle of silk strands, then approaches and injects its venom through the chelicerae or fangs, a pair of claws in the region of the mouth. In a few minutes, the struggle of the victim cease.

The spider prefers to reside in dim and remote haunts away from public notice.

The mother tincture is prepared from the whole spider.

Action of the Venom :

The venom of this spider is probably the most virulent as seen from the fact, that it has only about 1/200th of the amount of poison carried by the Prairie Rattler and yet it is about 15 times as potent.

The action of the venom is mainly neurotropic and is characterised by

- Generalised muscular cramps, spasms and rigidity.
- Sensation of constriction - 'Spider fetters its prey'.
- Haemorrhage of black blood.
- Slow vascular spasm at the extremities.
- Shivers, profuse cold sweat and pain which is very similar to angina pectoris.
- General pruritus.
- Desquamation of hands and feet.
- Sleeplessness. Restlessness.
- Mentally upset with a fear of going insane if a firm control is not exercised.
- Difficulty in breathing and talking.
- Slow action of the heart.

The crude provings of this venom was done by John Bradbury and Dr. A.W. Blair.

It was introudced into the Materia Medica by Jones and Tafel in 1889.

The venom causes interference to the passage of the nerve impulse at the neuromuscular junction where normal response depends on the release of acetylcholine. The venom causes premature release of all the acetylcholine, thus delaying the nerve impulse. But this is only a partial explanation of the biochemical effects of the venom.

Appearance of the Patient :

The patient has an expression of grave anxiety with extreme fear of dying and has a characteristic gait - bent forward with the hands held against the abdomen and the movement of the legs is achieved slowly and with difficulty. Speech may be difficult.

Miasm : Syphilitic.

Generals : It has an action on the heart causing a typical angina pectoris picture accompanied by restlessness and prostration.

General chilliness especially icy coldness of the extremities. Chilly but has flushes of heat.

Left sidedness.

Profuse perspiration.

Severe prostration but the patient cannot remain still due to great restlessness.

Extreme restlessness which does not allow the patient to sleep.

Pains - severe, constriction, cramping.

- come and go in waves, like labor pains.

Soreness of muscles especially to touch.

Haemorrhages - thin, watery blood.

Alcoholism.

Mind : (Corresponds to the feelings of a person facing death).

Extreme state of nervous irritation.

Fear of going mad.

Fear of losing breath and dying.

Fear of dying. Feels that death is approaching.

Sensitive to noise. Oversenstitiveness.

Restlessness. Constant tossing about. Ultimately mental prostration sets in, brainfag.

Shrieks, screams, moans, whines and shouts with pain.

Unrestrained and causeless crying in usually emotionally stable, strong men.

Head :

Occipital headache.

Constrictive, congestive pain.

< 2.50 - 3.00 P.M.

Mouth :

Lips cracked.

Tongue - white coated.
 - hyper-trophy of lingual papillae.
 - trembling
 - Increased salivation.

Increased thirst for cold water - vomits what he drinks. Appetite is ravenous or absent.

Stomach and Abdomen :

Sensation of pain or sinking at the epigastrium.

Nausea, vomiting of black blood which ameliorates.

Board like hardness of abdominal wall - No tenderness, but cramps on palpation.

Distension of abdomen is only slightly relieved by the passage of flatus.

Eructations.

Absolute inactivity of the rectum - Atony. Stools are black.

Respiratory System :

Dyspnoea, almost going into apnoea, slow laboured respiration with an uncontrollable expiratory grunt.

Difficulty in breathing due to muscle spasm.

Throat   - dry and congested
         - Pain on swallowing.

Cardio Vascular System :

Violent constrictive precordial pain extending to axilla and down the left arm, forearm to the tips of the fingers; with numbness and paresis of the affected limb.

Angina Pectoris - cramping pain from chest to abdomen.

Pulse   - Rapid
       - Upto 130 beats/minute
       - Weak, feeble, thready; almost impalpable.

Vascular hypotonia (or paradoxal hypertonia)
Hot flushes.
Swelling of ankles and puffiness of face.
< damp.

< before thunderstorm.

< night.

Urinary System :

Paralysis of Urinary bladder leading to retention of urine > by warm application, > sitting in a hot bath, > by puring warm water, over the perineum.

Urine   - Red, albuminous, with casts.
        - with burning.

Male :

Erections frequent

Testicular pain more on right side.

< movement.

Perspiration in the genital region.

Female :

Menstruation   - Suppressed
               - Scanty
               - Delayed.

Extremities :

Spastic paresis with increased reflexes.

Praresthesia of lower limb with difficulty in raising lower limbs because of spasm of hip extensor muscles. Tenderness of calf muscles on palpation.

Burning and stinging of soles of feet, as if they were on fire.

Tingling numbness of hands and feet.

Cramps from the nape to the loins.

Cramps, weakness.

Clonic spasms and trembling of whole body.

Back :

Shooting, cramping pains in lumbar region a feeling as if back was broken.

Skin :
    Increased hypersensitivity of skin.

    Soles of feet burn as if on fire.

    Icy cold - like marble; even in fever.

    Bluish skin.

    Cold perspiration.

    Formication - hypersensitivity of skin.

    Painful to touch in the lumbar, sacral region and hips and upper thighs.

Sleep :
    Anxious, disturbed

    Insomnia.

Dreams :
    Dreams of flying.

Modalities :

    < change of weather   > Hot bath

    < Damp   > Sitting quietly

    < Before thunderstorm.

    < Night

    < Alcohol

    < Exercise

    < Slightest movement, exertion.

Relationship :

    Compare Latrodectus Katipo and other Arachnida, Heloderma (coldness).

    Lach, Spig, Cimic., Cact., Kalm., Lycopus in Angina Pectoris.

LATRODECTUS MACTANS

Case :

Latrodectus Mactans, even though it is indicated for angina pectoris, I have used this remedy in a case of Carcinoma of the Bronchus with multiple bony metastasis where there was a sharp, shooting pain which used to come and go like waves. The patient was extremely chilly and restless with pain. Latrodectus Mactans 30 was used to reduce and palliate the complaints of the patient for long.

MYGALE LASIODORA COBANO

Source :

The source of this remedy is a large black live Cuban Spider.

Preparation :

It is prepared by putting the live black Cuban spider into alcohol.

It was first introduced and proved by Dr. J. C. Howard.

Crude Proving and Poisoning Effects :

It produces severe inflammation with green discoloration at the site of the bite and spreads along the lymphatics. Later the victim develops chill followed by fever, dryness of mouth, great thirst, trembling, dyspnoea and fear of death. There is also nausea, palpitation and severe stinging in urethra with hot scalding urine. It also produces twitchings and contractions of various muscies.

Clinical Utility :
* Chorea, especially of facial muscles (which is common to the order of Arachnida family).
* Chordee.
* Gonorrhoea.

Sphere of Action :
* Face
* Central Nervous System
* Genito Urinary Tract.

Symptomatology :

Generalities :
* Predominantly a right sided remedy.
* Tremulousness - constant motion of the whole body.
* Restlessness - constant motion especially of the hands and feet.
* Nervousness
* Red streaks along the lymphatics.

Mind : The characteristic mental state of Mygale is abrupt speech with restlessness, the patient is worse on waking. Like Bryonia, constantly talks of business with a strong fear of death. There are two polarities of extreme sensitivity on one end and feeling of hatred and revenge on the other.

Head :
* Jerking of head- more to right side
    - throwing the head backwards and forwads with a jerk.
* Dull frontal headache.

Face :
* Constant twitchings of the muscles of the face with mouth and eyes opening and closing in rapid succession.
* Constant contortions of face.
* Face hot and flushed.

Eyes :
   * Dimness of sight with nausea.

Ears :
   * Acute ear pain especially - right sided between midnight and morning.

Mouth :
   * Tongue - Dry, parched
            - Difficult to protrude
            - Coated brown.
   * Grating of teeth at night.
   * Speech difficult, jerking.

Stomach :
   * Nausea - with strong palpitations
            - with dimness of vision
            - with general weakness.
   * Appetite- decreased; more for dinner.
   * Aversion to food but > after eating.
   * Thirst excessive.

Urinary Organs :
   * Urine - increased, polyuria
           - hot, burning, scalding.
           - with stinging pain in urethra.

Male Sexualorgans :
   * Chordee
   * Protracted gonorrhoea
   * Syphilis
   * Violent erections in male.

Respiratory Organs :
  * Difficult breathing with desire for deep breaths.

Cardiovascular System :
  * Strong palpitations.
  * With concomittants   - nausea
                                        - vomiting
                                        - dimness of vision
                                        - chorea.

Back and Extermities :
  * Pain in the back extending around to the front.
  * Unsteady gait, dragging of feet while walking.
  * Constant motion of the whole body.
      - legs especially while sitting.
      - diffficult to keep hands in same position even for a minute.
  * Difficulty in carrying the hand to the mouth with jerking of hands either downwards or over the head or over the side of the face.
  * Uncontrollable convulsive movements of the arms and legs. Twitching and jerking of muscles of one arm and leg - usually right sided.
  * Limbs are quiet during sleep. Movements <

Skin :
  * Intense redness in streaks along the lymphatics from the calves upto the body.
  * Local inflammation reaching from the foot upto the knee leaves a large violet spot which later turns green.

Sleep
  * Restless all night with ridiculous dreams.

Fever :
 * Severe chill which lasts for half an hour; followed by fever with trembling of whole body, excessive thirst, flushed   face and dry coated tongue.

Modalities :   < eating
                   < sitting
                   < morning
                   > during sleep.

TARENTULA CUBENSIS

This spider also belongs to the family Lycosidae and is also known as the "Cuban Tarentula".

It is a large brown hairy spider found in Texas and South Carolina. There is an interesting history of this remedy as described by T.F. Allen. Tarentula Cubensis was being shipped to London in a container with alcohol to preserve it. On the way the container broke, the alcohol ran out and the specimen decomposed. However, a potency was made from this specimen and thus Tarentula Cubensis is a very important remedy for Carbuncles, abscesses, boils and swellings.

Generalities :

1. **Great sensitiveness with irritability :**
   Constant motion in the form of rubbing or fricition necessitates with this patient. This relieves the hyper irritation of the nervous system. They want to rub their hands and fingers with something hard for example - stick or against the wall.

2. **Periodicity :** Troubles occur at the same time every year.

3. Atrocious buring pains like Arsenic, Anthracinum.

4. Bluish discoloration of the affected part.

5. Great hyperaesthesia of female sexual system leading

to extreme sexual excitement.

Particulars :

Mind : Patient goes into delirium due to pain and sepsis.

Sympathetic, compassionate.

Head : Perspiration hot. Dull ache on top of the head. Dizziness after heat. Shooting pain through left eye across frontal region.

Mouth : Ulcers with marked burning, may spread to include the whole gastrointestinal tract (= Ars).

Stomach : Loss of appetite except for breakfast.

Urinary : Cannot hold urine on coughing. Retention. Intense pruritus vulvae.

Extremities : Hands tremble, turgid with blood. Feet restless. Tingling and numbness of tips of fingers.

Skin : Septic conditions of the skin. Red spots and pimples. Purplish hue. Burning, stinging pains. Gangrene. Abscesses, where pain and inflammation predominate. Senile ulcers. Paronychia.

Sleep : Sleep prevented by harsh cough. Cough > smoking. Sleep - restless. Drowziness.

Fever : Chills followed by intense burning fever with great thirst, anxiety, restlessness, headache, delirium, copious perspiration and retention of urine. Later the fever becomes intermittent accompanied by diarrhoea and prostration.

Modalities :   > Smoking.
                    < night.

Case of Tarentula Cubensis :

A 46 year old male came to me with a threatened gangrene of the dorsum of the right foot for which he had taken various treatment which did not yield.

It had started as a mosquito bite, and later developed into an abscess which burst open and discharged a brownish liquid. There was swelling of the foot with intolerable burning pain. The would had a lot of slough and redness. There was a sensation of numbness or heaviness of the ley with diminution of sensations.

Based on this picture Tarentula Cubensis was selected and administered in the 30th potency three times a day for 4 days. There was marked improvement of the wound - the burning pain, sweeling, discoloration and discharge all disappeared. The wound was healthy and healing, and the patient was more comfortable.

TARENTULA HISPANICA

Source : The spider from which this remedy is prepared is a species of wolf spider - LYCOSA TARENTULA. It is found mainly in Italy & Spain. Lycosa is a viscious looking creature with two large fangs and long legs which enable it to scurry rapidly in pursuit of its prey.

Poisoning effects :

The bite of the Tarentula is very painful and it produces a state called `Tarantulism' or `Tarantism' - the symptoms are either accompanied with or followed by an irresistible urge to dance with frenetic agitation.

The modern allopaths feel that `Tarantism' is not actually due to the poisonous effects of the venom but due to hysterical terror after being botten. Thus, whether a psychogenic factor is responsible based on fear and loathing, for the seizures of Tarantism, is still a controversy.

Various types of Tarantism were identified, the sporadic and the epidemic (particularly prevalent in the spring), the acute and the chronic (with relapses at the return of warm weather).

Tarantism, which was impossible to control could be suppressed and cured by music with a fast and strong rhythmic beat. The victims on hearing the music became excited and danced faster & faster till they fell down tired and sweating and got rid of the poison. This would last for 3 days.

Pharmacology :

Venom of this spider has affinity for the motor and sensory functions of the nervous system resulting in severe restlessness and uncontrolled agitation.

In the sensory sphere, there is excessive sensitivity and excitability of all' senses - light and glaring colurs irritate and aggravate. Also noise frightens and aggravates.

Affinity with the lymphatic and circulatory systems gives rise to cellulitis, lymphnode enlargement and vascular congestion, associated with facial pallor.

Proving : It was conducted and described by Marquis Nunez of Spain.

Doctrine of Signature :

1. Tarentula Hispania digs a vertical hole in the ground and covers it with a web so that it resembles the surroounding. Thus, it lures its unsuspecting prey. Such is the intelligence of this spider.

   Tarentula patients are also extemely intelligent to the extent of being foxy and cunning.

2. The Tarentula waits for its prey quiet and when the prey falls into its trap, it pounces on its prey with sudden and violent attacks and quickly goes back into the hole.

   This violence is seen in the Tarentula patient as violent movements like twitchings, jerkings and epilepsy. There is also tremendous amount of violence in the mental sphere which will be depicted in the next point.

3. The spiders are also well known for their Amatory dance. During the mating season, the male spider dances around the female spider. The female selects one and kills and eats away the others.

This is seen in the Tarentula patient as violence and destructiveness. These pts., are acute, quick acting (Hep, Stram, Tarent) can be very angry if contradicted. Their attacks can be quite aggressive. Though physically not very violent like Stram - they are verbally very aggressive - Rubic - threatening. Later on, they progress to tearing of clothes (Destructiveness of clothes), banging of head and other destructive states. Destructiveness - when he is being observed. Aversion to colours - red, black and green.

4. The spiders also use their web to communicate with each other. A long string connects the legs of two spiders - but it is very surprising as to why the spider does not get caught in its own web, since the strings are sticky. The reason for this is that, the spider creates two different types of strings - the spider always moves those set of strings which are not sticky. Thus, one can see the cunning nature of a spider.

The Tarentula pts. are very cunning. They know how to get what they want. They are great manipulators. Prone to lying and deception. Kleptomania, Feigning sickness. Tarentula pts. will often magnify their symptoms for secondary gain.

The pt. exhibits 'hysteria' or it is just a senstivity as in dislike of contradiction. Imagine that they have been insulted. Ailments from disappointed love or grief.

These pts. also exhibit hysteria on a sexual level.

Lascivious hysteria, Nymphomania can progress to shameful behaviour - exposes the person. They have increased desire for sex although it aggravates.

5. The hurried nature of the Tarentula patient is also attributed to the hurried activity in the nest of Tarentulas.

   Tarentula pts. feel compelled to move constantly and the lower extremeties are the most restless.

   Restlessness - bed, tossing about in. In the morning when he wakes up, the bed is in complete disarray.

   The restlessness is often coupled with anxiety. On the physical level, anxiety is found in the stomach, chest or region of the heart.

   The pts. have a feeling that something bad is going to happen or they are afraid things will not get done inspite of their hyperactivity.

   Tarentulas are hurried - they are annoyed if people in front of them walk slowly - hurry - everybody must. They walk very fast or will often run out of their restless compulsion.

   The industriousness also stems up from their need to diffuse all the energy in their bodies. They are very effective and highly productive in their work.

   The hurried nature of the pt. can also be attributed to the poison which hyperaccelerates the nervous system.

6. Tarentulas would annually migrate through a town named Tarantum (the spider got its name from this town). Thus pts. bitten by the spider have a return of symptoms every year at the same time (with decreasing violence). Thus, there is marked periodicity of symptoms.

TYPOLOGY :

Especially suited to mobile, restless people who cannot stay in one place and move constantly. The Tarantula type can be described as a woman with a changing, contradictory personality. She jumps from a state of happiness to melancholic sadness from calm and gentle behaviour to extreme violence.

Historical backgound :

In Southern Italy, large numbers of the 'Wolf Spider' would annually migrate through a town named tarantum and so the spider became named the 'Tarentula'. This spider was common to Mediterranean countries with a dry and sunny climate (Spain, Greece, Southern France, etc.)

The bite of this spider produced a convulsive condition, with an irresistible urge to dance known as tarantism. In many parts of Europe, there were may epidemics of convulsive dancing, in the 14th century. These epidemics spread rapidly and the outbreak became so serious that the church was obliged to resort to public exorcisms to drive out the devil. This dance in the latter part of the 17th century was still called the Lascivia chorea in German speaking countries. This dance in Italy was known since the 10th century and esp. in the South was attributed to the sting of Tarentula.

Towards the end of the 15th century, if was though that this dance was capable of actually curing a victim of the effects of the hypothetical poison of the Tarentula. The dance was stimulated by certain types of music and both the dance and the music of the Taranto region came to be known as `Tarentella'. This was at first a cure for

Tarantism and later developed into a dance of the upper class. The particupants were both men and women - men in thier powdered wigs and cod pieces, the women in masochistic corsets and caked rouge. Their dance was accompanied by fast music with a strong beat and a frenzied motion similar to Tarantism symtoms.

EVOLUTION OF TARENTULA MIND :
FROM THE PROVINGS :

1. The nervous system in Tarentula is would up tight like a coiled spring, tense with boundless energy which must be expended to prevent it from breaking. Thus, the Tarentula Patient is compelled to be busy, to act, to move without stopping. These are people in occupations requiring great responsibility and who are under tremendous pressure like journalist. They are industrious, capable, efficient but not due to ambition and competitiveness but due to sheer compulsion to keep busy.

    Because of the wound-up state of the nervous system, the tarentula Patient is relieved by soothing and calming influence of music. But the wrong kind of music furhter aggravates them.

2. All the other aspects of the mental state stem up from ill effects of unrequited love - the patient likes a girl very much but he has not spoken to her about his love. Thus, he will go out of his way to attract the girls attention - he wants to be noticed. He dances, wears colourful clothes to attract attention. He is cunning and mischevious.

3. In the second stage of illness, the patient loses control and becomes destructive. In such a state of tension, if the restless patient is restrained in some way, he becomes violent. At first, the destructiveness occurs only when the patient is alone, it is done secretly, hidden from others - cunningness of Tarentula. Later on, the destructiveness becomes more uncontrolled and publicly evident.

The third stage of pathology is characterised by insanity. On one hand ther is severe violence with desire to strike and kill and on the other hand, ther is an erotic mania in which the person makes overt sexual advances to other people and even to strangers.

The Tarentula activity is always very fast. Everything must be done quickly. He is very impatient, if other around him are slow. While walking too, the Tarentula Patient is always in a great hurry. This stems up not due a sense of anticipation but of a compulsion for rapid motion.

The Tarentual Patient is very anxious - anxiety that things will not get done, something will go wrong. The fear is usually irrational but it stems up from the wound-up state of the nervous system.

The Patients have a tendency to dance, to jump and to run and all these movements are rapid and vigorous movements. Tarentula patients are greatly aggravated from bright colours - red, yellow, green, black. There is marked hysteria in this remedy. This usually occurs when the external influences become too strong and the system collapses. There may be spasms, fainting attacks, convulsive states.

TARENTULA
(From the Repertory)

Mind : To study the mind of Tarentula, one learns quite a lot by observing the patient in the clinic. As soon as he enters the clinic he just roams around the corridor.
- ANXIETY, causeless.
- Busy, fruitless
- HURRY, haste
  They are usually dressed in bright colours to attract the attention.
- COLOURS charmed by blue, green, red.
  Whenever a question is asked to them by the physician either they do not follow or .....
- ABSENTMINDED, unobservant
- ANSWERS, questioned, does not answer, when
- ANSWER, aversion to
- ANSWER, refuses to
- UNDERSTAND questions addressed to her does not
..... if at all they answer - very abruptly, curtly and shortly.
- ANSWER, abrupt.
  During the interview they are quite inattentive ....
- CONCENTRATION, difficult, conversation during.
- or when they are sitting in front of the physician, they make various gestures.
- GESTURES, grasping, fingers in the mouth, children put
- GESTURES, grasping, hands restlessly busy.
- GESTURES, nervous
- GESTURES, plays with his fingers.
- GESTURES, wringing the hands
- PULL, one's hair desire to
- SCRATCHES with hands.

It the patient is a child, he is extremely restless, will touch various things kept on the physician's table. They usually detest being examined.
- JUMPING
- MISCHIEVIOUS
- RESTLESSNESS, anxious.
- ANGER, when touched
- FEAR, of touch
- LOOKED AT, cannot bear to be
- PRESENCE OF STRANGERS, aggravates.

If the parents scold them, they are completely indifferent or they retaliate and may become violent, tear their clothes, pull their hair or they have a habit of hiding and their parents have to search for them.
- ANGER, violent
- BITES, himself
- KICKS
- RUNS about
- STRIKING, anger from
- CONTRARY
- HIDE, desire to

Surprisingly, they may behave so nicely and leave such a good impression on the physician, that many a times the physician feels that the parents are giving an exactly opposite description.
- IMPRESSIONABLE.

Sometimes when they are out of control, the parents have to hit them. This increases their violence tremendously
—RAGE, pulls hair of bystanders.
- STRIKING, head his
- STRIKING, himself.

- STRIKING, strikes her head with her hands, her body and others.
- TEARS, hair, her things.
  The same child when he grows into an adult, they are extremely restless, always in a hurry. They must be in constant motion, even though motion aggravates. They have boundless energy which compels them to be busy.
  In an office, they always want their colleagues to hurry as they always feel that people do their work slowly. The same thing is manifested at the physical level e.g., hands are in constant motion, constant motion of the leg, ludicrous motion of arms and trunk.
- ACTIVITY, fruitless
- ACTIVITY, mental
- GESTURES, grasping or reaching at something, at flocks; carphologia.
- GESTURES, involuntary (motion hands) knitting, as if
- GESTURES, makes
- GESTURES, ridiculous or foolish.
- IMPULSE run to, dromomania.
- INDUSTRIUS, mania for work.
- MUSIC, ameliorates, restlessness of extremities.
- RESTLESSNESS, 5 h.
- RESTLESSNESS, anxious, compelling rapid walking.
- RESTLESSNESS, bed, go from one bed to another, wants to
- RESTLESSNESS, bed, tossing about in
- RESTLESSNESS, menses during
- RESTLESSNESS, driving about
- RESTLESSNESS, music from
- HURRY, everybody must hurry,
- HURRY movements in
- HURRY walking while

- IMPATIENCE
  There patients are guided by whims. They are extremely sly and cunning having fear to face real opposition. Dr. Margaret Tyler in her drug pictures mentions about sudden violence what she calls as "unexpected behaviour." This cunning behaviour is characterised by destructive movements.
- CRAFTY
- DECEITFUL, sly
- DESTRUCTIVENESS, cunning
- FEIGNING, paroxysms, faintness
- FEIGNING, sick
- WEEPING, hysterical
- DESTRUCTIVENESS, clothes of
- MANIA, destruction, followed by laughter and apologies, of paroxysmal.
- RAGE, fury
- SHRIEKING, screaming, shouting.
- TEARS hair, and presses her head.
- THREATENING, destroy, threatens to.
- THREATENING, kill, threatens to
- THROWS, things away.
- VIOLENT, deeds of violence, rage leading to.
  They have extreme disposition to laugh, play, joke and to do absurd things.
- CHEERFUL, gay, mirthful
- DANCING, wild
- ECCENTRICITY
- EXCITEMENT, music from
- EXCITEMENT, dancing, singing and weeping with
- EXHILARATION
- EXTROVERT (people)
- FOOLISH, behaviour

- INSANITY, laughing with
- JESTING
- JESTING, walking on
- LAUGHING, company in
- LAUGHING, desire to laugh
- LAUGHING, immoderately
- LAUGHING, involuntarily
- LAUGHING, mocking
- LAUGHING, nervous
- LAUGHING, sardonic
- LAUGHING, screams, then
- LAUGHING, stupid expression, with
- LOQUACITY
- MANIA, singing with
- MOOD, changeable, variable
- PLAYFUL
- SHRIEKING, laughter, after
- SINGING, dancing and weeping
- SINGING, hoarse until very, exhausted and
- SINGING, involuntarily
- VIVACIOUS
- VIVACIOUS, alternating sorrow with.

Leading Symptoms :

1. **Extreme restlessness :** The patient must be in constant motion, though motion aggravates. Desire to jump. Boundless energy. Compelled to be busy, to act.

   Hyperactivity, rapid movement. Hands and legs in constant motion. Tries to work his overexcitability but lacks control.

2. **Sensitive to music :** Better by music, rhythm, (massaging, riding on horseback, smoking) and dancing. Even physically affected by colour.

3. **Chilly** yet desire for, and better in open air.

4. **Twitchings** : The nerves are highly strung. Jerking. Starting from sleep. Restless hands, legs.

5. **Sexual Erethism** : Sensitive genitals.

6. **Aversion** : Meat, bread, chocolate.

7. **Desire** : Spicy food, sand, cold drinks, highly seasoned food, salty things, lime, raw food, sand and ash. (They scrape the burnt food from bottom of vessel).

8. **Hysterical disposition** : Feign sickness, worse when observed, better when alone. Sudden changes in mood. Fainting, twitching, choking. Selfish, hateful, foxy, cunning, strange fancies with regard to colours. Violence. Throws things, pulls hair, destructive. Aversion to red, green black and all striking colours. Desire to lie down in the dark and not to be talked to. Angered from contradiction.

9. **Periodicity of compaints** : Some complaints occur at the, same hour or at the same period annually.

10. **Right sided affections** : Involvement of the left arm and right leg. (Opposite to Agaricus)

11. **Hyperaesthesia** : Of skin, genitals, eyes (Photophobia), finger tips (needle like sensation).

PARTICULARS :

Head :* Headache as if "a thousand needles were pricking the brain."
   * Sensation "as if cold water was being poured on the head and over the body."
   * Constantly rolls his head, back and forth on the pillow (Bell, Hell).
   < by stooping

> rubbing the head against the pillow.
< contact or touch
< after study
< walking
< towards evening.
* Vertigo. Wants hair to be brushed or rubbed.
* Concomittant - Photophobia.

Eyes : * Loss of vision in right eye.
* Right pupil may be enlarged and left contracted.
* Pain is felt in right eye.
* Vision may be dim.
* Sensation of foreign body in the eye - eyelash, splinter, sand.

Ears : * Cracking may occur in the right ear, associated with pain and hiccough.
* Tinnitus is present at night < on walking.
   as of ringing of bells.

Nose : * Epistaxis > throbbing carotids and fullness in head.

Alimentary System :
* Dryness of mouth and teeth.
* Strawberry tongue (Bell, Frag)
* Throbbing toothache < breathing in air.
* Fauces - swollen, purple.
          - tonsils inflammed and large to obstruct breathing.
* Sensation of constriction when swallowing.
* Nausea, acidity, burning pain in stomach < by drinking water.
* Sensation as if "something alive was moving in or causing tingling in stomach and rising up to the throat."

* Diarrhoea - Profuse
- with nausea, vomiting, fainting and prostration.
- stools - dark, very offensive.
- pain and burning of anus after stools.

Respiratory System :
* Cough - dry, spasmodic
- with retching and gagging.
- with involuntary urine.
- < evening > smoking.
- causes pain in head, chest and uterus.
* Chronic coryza - with frequent sneezing.
- chiefly affects the right nostril.
* Epistaxis - Profuse, dark, quickly coagulating blood.
* Chest - great oppression with panting respiration.
* Suffocation with crying, screaming and restlessness.

Cardiovascular System :
* Precordial anxiety with tumultuous palpitation.
* Angina and Mitral Valve disease.
* Sensation af if the heart was being squeezed or compressed or was turning and twisting.
* Cannot lie on the left side.
* < Putting hands in cold water.

Lymphatic System :
* Cervical lymphadentiis with tonsillitis may cause such severe swelling of the neck so as to endanger life from obstruction to breathing.

Urinary System :
* Cystitis with excruciating pain and acute retention.

* Dysuria, Polyuria with frequent and very painful urination < at night.
* Incontinence on laughing, coughing, sneezing.
* Diabetes Mellitus.
* Drawing pain in urethra < after urinating.
* Spasmodic urinary retention.
* Albumen in urine.

Genital System :
* Male* Libido is increased.
      * Testicular tumours - indolent.
      * Lasciviousness reaching almost to insanity. < Coition.
      * Sensitive genitals.
      * Prostatic ailments after masturbation.
* Female : * Nymphomania. < coitus.
      * Violent itchng of the genitals < after menses.
      * Pruritus as if insects crawling.
      * Fibroid tumours. Cancer of cervix.
      * Bearing down feeling as of a great weight in the pelvis with uterine pain and burning in hypogastrium and hips.
      * Menses - early, profuse, followed by severe pruritus vulvae.
      * During menses - intolerable dryness of nose, throat, tongue and mouth.
      * Cramps after abortion.

Locomotor System :
      * Keeps hand in constant motion, constant motion of legs; ludicrous motion of arms and trunk. Picks fingers.
      * Weakness of legs as if dead.
      * Numbness of parts.
      * Twitching and jerking, trembling.

* Yawning with uneasiness of legs, must move them constantly.
* Temperature subnormal.
* Sensation of crawling of insects.
* Can run better than walk.
* Rigidity and muscle cramps with extreme weakness and paresis presumably due to involvement of spinal cord.
* Chorea > music or < music. Chorea only when someone is watching.
* Restless limbs < evening, in bed before.

Skin : * A variety of eruptions with - purpuric sports, vesicular or miliary eruptions.
* Pruritus extreme, sensation of formication, burning, scorching, numbness, excessive hyperaesthesia especially at the finger tips.
* Carbuncle, Deep abscesses. Helps evacuation of pus.
* Dry eczema, itching as of insects creeping and crawling.
* Cold spots or as of a cold matter flowing or dropping on part.

Sleep: * Sleepless from excitement before midnight.
* Dreams sad; with weeping.

Modalities :
< or > music.
< any strong emotion (grief, excitement).
< cold, damp weather, exposure to cold air.
< when walking; yet cannot keep still.
< from noise.
< light touch.
< by wetting hands in cold water.

< Bright light.
< When at rest.
< at night.
< after coitus.
< washing head.
> Dry sunny days, in the sun.
> Open air (though vertigo is aggravated out of doors)
> warm room.
> From firm pressure; friction; rubbing.
> After a nose bleed.
> Dancing.

Tarentula

Relations

Antidote to : Lach (Herring), Partial antidotes : Puls, Mag-C, Mosch, Cupr, Chel, Gels, Bov, Carb. Veg.

Compare -
- Desire to jump - Stram, Croc, Nat-m, Stict, Asar, Agar, Hyos, Cic.
- Hysteria, alternation of moods, sensation of something alive, black, clots, epistaxis - Croc.
- Unfortunate love - Ph-ac.
- Nymphomania - Cann-i, Canth, Hyos, Murex, Orig, Phos, Verat-a.
- Music aggravates - Acon, Ambr, Graph, Nat-c, Nux-v., Sabin, Sep. Thuja.
- Fear of touch or contact - Acon, Ant-c, Arn, Bell, Cham, Cina, Cinch, Colch, Hep-s, Kali-c, Lach, Nux.v, Plb., Spig.
- Hysteria - Ambr, Asaf, Cimic, Cocc, Croc, Gels, Ign, Kali-p, Mosch, Nux-m, Phos, Plat, Puls, Sep, Samb, Valer, Zinc-val.

- Loquacity - Agar, Cimic, Hyos, Lach, Stram.
- Desires to do absurd things - Bell, Cic, Hyos, Stram.
- Laughs immoderately at trifles - Anac, Cann-i, Croc, Hyos, Mosch, Plat, Stram.
- Sing - Agar, Croc, Hyos, Stram.
- Tears things - Bell, Cimex, Stram, Verat-a.
- Aimlessly busy - Arg-n, Lit-t.
- Cruel, inhuman, violent - Anac, Croc, Nil-ac, Nux-v, Plat, Stram, Verat-a.
- Rubbing ameliorates - Canth, Mag-p, Phos, Podo.
- Very sensitive to noise, slightest noise startles from sleep - Asar, Calad, Nux-v.
- Mania with desire to cut and tear things esp. clothes - Verat-a.
- Oversensitivity of nerves, scratching of linen or silk, crackling of paper is unbearable - Asar, Ferr-m, Nit-ac, Nux-v., Ther.
- Restlessness - anxious - Ars, Kali-ar., Kali-c, Nat-a, Nat-c.
- Hurry - Lit-t, Med., Merc, Nat-m, Sulph, Sul-ac.
- Hurry movements in - Stram, Sulph-ac.
- Hurry - walking, while - Arg-n, Sulph-ac.
- Hurry - everybody must hurry - Arg-n, Cann-i, Lach, Nat-p., Nux-m.
- Destructiveness of clothes - Bell, Camph, Hyos, Ign, Nux-v, Plb., Stram, Sulph, Verat.
- Anger, violent - Acon, Anac, Aur, Cham, Hep, Nit-ac, Nux-v, Staph.
- Anger, touched when - Ant-c, Iod.
- Dancing - Acon, Agar, Apis, Bell, Cann-i, Carc, Cic, Cocc, Con, Croc, Crot-t, Hyos, Ign, Merc, Nat-m, Ph-ac, Pip-m, Plat, Rob, Santin.
- Insanity - Ars, Bell Hyos, Lyc, Merc. Nux-v., Stram, Verat.

- Insanity - Strength increased - Agar, Bell, Canth, Corr-r, Hyos, Stram.
- Threatening - Agar, Hep, Stam, Tub, Valer.
- Work - desire for mental - Anth, Aloe, Arn, Bad, Brom, Carb-ac, Chin, Clem, Cob, Coca, Eug, Ham, Lach, Laur, Naja, Nat-m, Nat-p, Ped, Pip-m, Rhus-t, Seneg, Sulph, Samb, Ther.
- Industrious - Aur, Tub.
- Hysteria - Asaf, Aur, Caust, Cocc, Con, Gels, Ign, Kali-p, Lach, Mag-m, Nat-m, Nit-ac, Nux-m, Nux-v, Plat, Puls, Sep., Sil, Valer, Verat.
- Disobedience - Acon, Agn, Am-c, Am-m, Arn, Calc, Canth, Caps, Caust, Chin, Dig, Elae, Guaj, Lyc, Merc. Nit-ac, Nux-v, Petr., Phos Spig, Staph, Sulfonal Sulph, Viol-o, Viol-t.
- Obstinate - Alum, Anac, Arg-n, Bell, Calc, Cham, Nux-v, Tub.
- Contrary - Alum, Anac, Arg-n, Lach, Merc.
- Fear - walking of rapidly.
- Feigning sick - Arg-n, Bell, Ign, Plb, Sabad, Sil, Verat.
- Sensitive noise to, music, amel - Aur.
- Touched, aversion to being - Ant-c, Cham, Kali-c.
- Dancing - Acon, Aether, Agar, Apis, Bell, Cann-i, Carc, Chiol, Cic., Cocc., Con., Croc., Crot-t, Grat, Hyos, Ign., Merc., Nat-m, Phos-ac, Pip-m., Plat., Rob, Santin, Sep., Sil., Stict., Stram, Tab.

Compare :
- Irritation of periphery of neves exercising, rubbing - Kali-br.
- Chorea - Mygal, Cimic, Agar, Stram.
- Bores head into pillow - Bell, Hell.
- Fidgety feet - Caust, Zinc.
- Periodicity of complaints - Aran, Ars., Cact, Cinch, Eup-per, Ign, Nat-m, Tela.

- · Periodicity every year - Ars., Carb-v., Crot-hor, Lach, Sulph, Thuja.
- Aggravation at rest - Arn., Ars, Cycl, Ferr-m, Merc, Puls, Rhod, Rhus-t, Samb, Sep.
- Restlessness - Acon, Agar, Ars, Bapt Bell, Cham, Cimic, Coff, Ign., Rhus-t., Sulph.
- Jerkings, twitchings, starting during sleep, - Acon, Aeth, Agar, Apis, Bell, Cina, Hyos, Ign, Lyc, Stam, Sulph, Zinc-m.
- Restlessness - Acon, Anac, Arg-n, Ars, Ars-i, Bapt., Bell, Calc., Calc-p, Camph, Cimic, Cit-v, Coloc, Cup Cupr-ar, ferr, Ferr-ar, Hyos, Lyco, Merc Plb, Puls, Pyrog, Rhust-t, Sec., Sep, Sil, Staph, Stram, Sulph, Zinc.
- Restlessness - bed - tossing about in - Ars., Cupr., Ferr, Ip, Rhust.
- Restlessness anxious compelling rapid walking - Ars.

TARENTULA HISPANICA
Tarentula hispanica has been used by me in the following cases very frequently :
* Bedwetting.
* Epilepsy
* Behavioural problems
* Severe constipation

Summing up the common symptoms on which Tarentula hispanica has been indicated.
* > music
* Restlessness
* Violence
* Desires raw food
* Obstinate, when refused lied on ground and bange the head.
* Hot patient

* Mischievious
* Jealous
* Loves dancing

It is very interesting to note that Stramonium. Tarentula and Tuberculinum come very close in pediatric case prescription.

Case of Tarentula Hispanica :

One morning at about 4 a.m., a lady came home desperately asking for help. Her father-in-law had not passed stools since two days inspite of giving three enemas.

When I went to her house, I saw an 80 year old man, in messed up clothes, shouting fearfully that he was going to die.

While his son started to give me the history, he abused him and said that it was he who was sick and that he would give the history himself. He said that he had a sensation as if there was a machine gun in his rectum. He had a feeling that everything was packed inside.

On examining him, I found two deep fissures which caused the inability to pass the stool. The following rubrics were taken :
* Constipation, stool remains in rectum, with awful anxiety.
* Anxiety hypochondriacal.
* Answers abruptly, shortly.
* Anger violent.
* Anxiety, health about.
* Abusive.

Tarentula hispanica 200 single dose was given. In two hours the pain decreased and the patient could pass stool. The patient felt much better and no medicine was required thereafter.

THERIDION CURASSAVICUM

Source : Orange spider - The spider is found in the West Indies, chiefly in the island of Curagoa. It is about the size of a cherry stone and is found on orange trees. The spider is velvety black when young, with antero posterior lines composed of white dots, on posterior part of the body there are three orange-red spots and a large square yellow spot on the belly. It is very poisonous. The spider belongs to the family Argelenidae.

Pharmacology : The poison produces a highly sensitive, nervous condition with weakness, trembling, coldness, anxiety, faintness and easily excited cold sweat. There is marked affinity for the bony structures as well as to the nervous organs they enclose. It produces auditory hyper-sensitivity and dizziness.

Proving : It was introduced and proved by Herring in 1832. The alcoholic tincture is prepared from crushed live spiders.

Appearance : It acts most effectively on nervous, hypersensitive people who feel that time passes to quickly.

Psychology : Marked oversensitivity to noise (Noises causes nausea, vertigo, chills, and pains all over; seems to penetrate the body.

Time appears to pass rapidly, although he does little. Despair; want of self confidence. Tries to occupy himself constantly, but finds pleasure in nothing.

Inclined to be startled (Startled by least things)
Talkative after spirituous beverages.

Symptomatogy Every shrill sound penetrates the body.

General : Theridion is most often a remedy, for women. When we find the combination of vertigo, insomnia and tremendous oversensitivity to noise, Theridion is the remedy.
Extremely chilly patient.
Extreme sensitiveness during puberty, during pregnancy and climacteric years.
Most complaints are accompanied by vertigo.
Closing the eyes aggravate, (Nausea and vertigo)
Sea sickness.
Bones seem broken (rickets, caries, necrosis of bones).
Pain in all the bones. Weakness, Coldness in body parts. Tetanus with trismus; has an affinity for the tubercular diathesis.

Head :
Vertigo :
< closing eyes   Vertigo with nausea (Lach)
< Motion   Vertigo with headache.
< riding in a carHysterical Vertigo.
< Noise
< Sleep on going to
< Sleep after
< Turning on.

Headache :
Location : Forehead extends to the occiput
        Eyes - behind - (L) eye.
Occiput

Sensation : Band like at the root of the nose
Pulsating.
< closing on, eyes
< Noise
< Noise from rattling of vehicles (Nitric acid)
< heat of sun
< lying down - must sit or walk
Sunstroke

Eyes : Sensitive to light, Objects look double. Dull pressure behind eyes < closing eyes. Nausea, vomiting, vertigo < closing eyes. Throbbing over left eye.
Luminous vibrations before eyes.

Ears : Least noise < Every shrill sound penetrates the body, esp., teeth, < vertigo; cannot bear loud noises rushing in ears like a waterfall, with impaired hearing. Roaring in ears.

Nose : Thick, yellowish green offensive discharge from nose. Ozaena. Pressure in root of nose and heaviness. Sneezing in evening, with coryza.

Face : Face-pale. Jaw unmovable in morning on waking; and at other timed of the day, then opening involuntarily.

Teeth : Every shrill sound penetrates the teeth. Sensation as if cool water were too cold.
Biting of tongue - sleep during.

Stomach : Craving for oranges & bananas. Increased desire to smoke tobacco. Thirst for wine and brandy. Nausea, vomitting < closing eyes and, motion seasickness. Stinging pain on left side over anterior aspect of spleen. Burning in liver region. Desires dry rice. Aversion to meat. Nausea after cold drinks.

Rectum : Spasmodic contraction of rectum and anus. Stools-papescent. Scanty, urgent. stool difficult towards the end, though not hard.

Respiratory : Pain in upper left chest. Pain in left floating ribs. Pinching in left pectoral muscles. Violent cough with *spasmodic jerking of head forwards and knees upwards.*

Heart : Cardiac anxiety and pain. Pain radiates to arm and left shoulder. Pulse slow with vertigo.

Back : Sensitiveness between vertebrae. Stinging pains, *sits sideways* in a chair *to avoid pressure* against spine.
Spinal irritation. Curvature of spine in growing girls.

Skin : Hard pimple beside ball of thumb. Itching stinging thrusts everywhere.

Sleep : Sleepy in the morning. Deep sleep at night. He often bites tip of his tongue during sleep. Dreams of journey in distant regions and of riding on horses. Dreams that he broke off a tooth.

Fever : Shaking chill with foam at mouth with headache and vomiting. Icy sweat covering body with fainting, vertigo and vomiting at night.

Modalities : Ailments from sea travelling, riding, washing clothes.

Aggravation : Touch
Pressure,
riding in a carriage or ship
jar, noise
coitus
left side

Clinical conditions
Auditory hyperasthesia
Menieres disease
Rickets, caries, necrosis.
Curvature of spine
In scrofula, where the best selected remedies fail
to relieve.

Relations : Antidoted by Aconite (Sensitiveness to noise)
Mosch (Nausea)
Graph (More chronic effects)
Remedies that precede well - Sulph, Calc-c Lyc.

Comparision : Hemicrania, worse from closing eyes &
noise - Sep. Vertigo & faintness worse closing eyes
- Lach, Thuja Cannot bear scratching of line, silk
or crackling of paper - Asar, Ferr-m, Tarax.
Time passes too slowly - Arg-n, Cann-i, Nux-m,
Glon.
Time passes too quickly - Cocc.
Nasal cattarh; thick, yellow or greenish offensive
Puls, Thuj.
Headache < lying down - Lach.
Bites tongue in sleep - Ph-ac (bites sides)
Theri (bites tip)
Effect of washing clothes - Phos.

Case 1

An old lady with Multi infact dementia presented with
vertigo and insomnia. Vertigo was accompanied with
nausea and was worse on going to sleep. In order to avoid
work, this patient would feign and have hysterical
symptoms and make her children do all the work.
The following symptoms were selected to prescribe
Theridion :
* Hysteria.
* Vetigo, closing eyes on, nausea with.

*   "   motion from, vomiting and nausea.
*   "   nausea with.
*   "   nausea with, closing eyes on.
*   "   sleep during.
*   "   sleep on going to.
*   "   sleeping after aggravates.
*   "   vomiting with.
* Sleeplessness, midnight before.
* Sleeplessness, vertigo from.
* Waking, nausea from.
* Waking, vertigo from.

Few does of Theridion 30 were prescribed on the above rubrics and fair improvement was seen in the condition of the patient.

Case 2

A 76 years old Parsi woman, suffering from sinusitis - Bronchitis (C.O.P.D.) and Osteo arthritis was being treated with Phosphorus. In general, she had improved a lot in her complaints except for Vertigo.

After going through the full case and past follow-ups, I collected the symptoms she had given with the complaint of Vertigo, and they were as follows :

* Vertigo < at night.
* Vertigo always associated with insomnia.
* Patient wakes up from sleep because of vertigo, sometimes full night is very restless because of vertigo.
* Giddiness < movements of head.
* Heaviness of left frontal region of head.

Initially Theridion 30 was given twice a day and patient showed considerable improvement but later there was a status quo, hence the potency was stepped up to 200 and the patient showed improvement by 80%. Still, the patient is on Theridion.

DREAMS OF SPIDERS

(1) **Tarentula hispanica**
- Animals
- Animals - wild
- animals - pursuing him
- Bulls - pursuing him
- Business
- Contempt
- Danger
- Dead bodies
- Death
- Horse - falling from horse
- Insults (abused)
- Long
- Many (dreaming)
- Misfortune (accidents, disaster, events, unfortunate, loss)
- Pleasant (joyous, peaceful, quiet, wonderful)
- Pleasant after 2 h.
- Pursued being animals by
- Pursued, being, bulls by
- Remembered
- Sad (cares, weeping)
- Unpleasant (disgusting)

- Unremembered
- Vexations (anger, quarrel, upleasant, striving)
- Water (bathing, danger, drowning, falling, fishes, flood, journey, jumping, rowing, sailing, sea, stream, storm, wading, walking).

(2) Theridion

- Body parts of - teeth breaking off
- Disease - teeth breaking off
- Horses
- Horse riding
- Journeys (difficulties, foreign country)
- Journeys horse back, on
- Many
- Riding
- Teeth - breaking off

(3) Mygale

Absurd (strange)

Ludicrous

(4) Aranea Diadema

Frightful (anxious)

COMMON THEME OF DREAMS OF SPIDERS

As mentioned earlier in the chapter of evolution of mind the dreams of spiders basically suggest a threat to the person from the environment. Since the person has engaged himself in many unsocial activities he faces a constant stress in the subconscious mind in the form of dreams, e.g.

Dreams of animals

Dreams of animals wild

Dreams of animals pursuing him

Dreams of Bulls Pursuing him

Dreams of Danger

Dreams of Horse falling from a horse

Dreams of pursued being animals by

Dreams of pursued being, bulls by

Further being pursued by a bull often shows the frustration arising from the basic drives being taunted or thwarted; for instance a person - may wish for family yet be frustrated by a from of sexuality in their partner which does not care for the instinctive drive for children.

Similarly, falling from a horse indicated pleasurable energy and exhuberance with dynamic sexual drive.

Losing the teeth, indicates the aging process as it relates to maturity. This is because we lose our first teeth as a we leave childhood behind, and lose our adut teeth as we leave youthfulness behind.

As one studies Theridion, one gathers an impression that it is chiefly used in complaints of the old. For example, it is useful for tubercular affection of the bones - caries, necrosis and pthisis of lungs, prostatic hypertrophy, gonorrhoea and liver abscess. It is also useful where the indicated remedy does not hold long.

All the above indicates an advanced chronic condition, in elderly individuals, hence the dream of teeth breaking off.

BIBLIOGRAPHY

* Agrawal, M.L. Materia Medica of the Human Mind.
* Barthel, H. Synthetic Repertory Vol. I, II, III.
* Bhanja, K.C. Masterkey to Homoeopathic Materia Medica.
* Boericke, William Materia Medica with Repertory.
* Desmond Morris - Animal Watching.
* Gibson, Douglas M. Studies of Homoeopathic Remedies.
* Kent, J.T. Lectures on Homoeopathic Materia Medica.
* Kent, J.T. Repertory of the Homoeopathic Materia Medica.
* Michael Chinery - Life Story - Spider.
* Murphy, Robin Fundametals of Materia Medica.
* Phatak, S.R. Materia Medica of Homoeopathic Medicines.
* Sankaran, Rajan Tarentula Hispanica - A Study.

BOOKS BY THE SAME AUTHOR

1. Medicine in Mnemonics
2. Forensic Medicine in Mnemonics
3. Bed-wetting (Enuresis)
4. A Patient's Guide to Homoeopathy
5. Homoeopathy in Epilepsy
6. Perceiving Rubrics of Mind
7. The Disease of Skin
7. Hair Loss
8. Cancer
9. Sycotic Shame
10. Mysterious Thuja
11. Mr. Lycopodium
12. Homoeopathy Lactose Intolerance
13. St. Ignatius Bean
14. Tubercular Miasm-Tuberculines
15. Bach Flower Rem. for Everyone